DMSO Book

A Beginner's Overview on its Use Cases for Inflammatory Conditions, with a Potential 6-Step Plan

copyright © 2025 Patrick Marshwell

All rights reserved No part of this book may be reproduced, or stored in a retrieval system, or transmitted in any form or by any means, electronic, mechanical, photocopying, recording, or otherwise, without express written permission of the publisher.

Disclaimer

By reading this disclaimer, you are accepting the terms of the disclaimer in full. If you disagree with this disclaimer, please do not read the guide.

All of the content within this guide is provided for informational and educational purposes only, and should not be accepted as independent medical or other professional advice. The author is not a doctor, physician, nurse, mental health provider, or registered nutritionist/dietician. Therefore, using and reading this guide does not establish any form of a physician-patient relationship.

Always consult with a physician or another qualified health provider with any issues or questions you might have regarding any sort of medical condition. Do not ever disregard any qualified professional medical advice or delay seeking that advice because of anything you have read in this guide. The information in this guide is not intended to be any sort of medical advice and should not be used in lieu of any medical advice by a licensed and qualified medical professional.

The information in this guide has been compiled from a variety of known sources. However, the author cannot attest to or guarantee the accuracy of each source and thus should not be held liable for any errors or omissions.

You acknowledge that the publisher of this guide will not be held liable for any loss or damage of any kind incurred as a result of this guide or the reliance on any information provided within this guide. You acknowledge and agree that you assume all risk and responsibility for any action you undertake in response to the information in this guide.

Using this guide does not guarantee any particular result (e.g., weight loss or a cure). By reading this guide, you acknowledge that there are no guarantees to any specific outcome or results you can expect.

All product names, diet plans, or names used in this guide are for identification purposes only and are the property of their respective owners. The use of these names does not imply endorsement. All other trademarks cited herein are the property of their respective owners.

Where applicable, this guide is not intended to be a substitute for the original work of this diet plan and is, at most, a supplement to the original work for this diet plan and never a direct substitute. This guide is a personal expression of the facts of that diet plan.

Where applicable, persons shown in the cover images are stock photography models and the publisher has obtained the rights to use the images through license agreements with third-party stock image companies.

Table of Contents

Introduction	6
What Is DMSO?	9
Industrial Use	10
How Does DMSO Work?	11
Different Types of DMSO	15
Different Forms of DMSO and Their Uses	18
Use Cases of DMSO	22
Pros and Cons of DMSO	27
Pros of Using DMSO	27
Cons	29
Potential Side Effects of DMSO	30
Potential Step-by-Step Guide To Get Started with DMSO	33
Step 1: Consultation	33
Step 2: Choosing the Right Concentration	39
Step 3: Preparation	43
Step 4: Application Method	48
Step 5: Monitoring and Adjusting	53
Step 6: Long-term Considerations	61
Best Practices for Maximizing Benefits and Minimizing Risks	69
Safety Precautions and Consideration for DMSO Usage	72
Dosage Instructions	72
Adverse Effects	73
Precautions and Warnings	73
Common Mistakes to Avoid	75
Things to Do and to Avoid When Using Dimethyl Sulfoxide (DMSO)	76
Things to Avoid	77
Conclusion	79
FAQs	82
References and Helpful Links	84

Introduction

Dimethyl sulfoxide, commonly known as DMSO, may not be a household name, but its applications span various fields from medical treatments to industrial uses. Originating as a byproduct of paper manufacturing, this colorless liquid has been recognized for its ability to penetrate biological membranes and has gained attention for some of its unique properties.

You might be wondering what exactly makes DMSO an intriguing substance worth exploring. The story of DMSO is rich with scientific investigations, medical anecdotes, and a fair share of controversies. Some hail it as a versatile remedy with potential benefits ranging from pain relief to anti-inflammatory effects, while others caution against its use due to possible side effects and lack of comprehensive research.

Understanding DMSO's multifaceted nature requires delving into its chemical properties, mechanisms of action, and the contexts in which it is used. Whether you're considering its use for personal health reasons or simply curious about its scientific background, this guide aims to provide a balanced view, ensuring you are informed about both its potential and its risks.

In this guide, you will learn about the following:

- What is DMSO?
- How Does DMSO Work?
- Different Types and Forms of DMSO
- Use Cases of DMSO
- Pros and Cons of DMSO
- Step-by-Step Guide To Get Started with DMSO
- Safety Precautions and Consideration for DMSO Usage

Equipping yourself with knowledge about DMSO will help you make informed decisions. This guide does not advocate for or against its use but rather seeks to present the information neutrally, so you understand the precautions necessary if you decide to explore DMSO further.

As you progress through this guide, we encourage you to approach DMSO with an open mind and a critical perspective. Always consider consulting with healthcare providers before using any new substance, particularly one as potent and under-researched as DMSO. Our aim is to ensure that if you decide to explore the use of DMSO, you can do so in a safe and responsible manner.

By the end of this guide, you'll have a well-rounded understanding of DMSO, empowering you to make decisions based on evidence and careful consideration. Keep reading for an informative journey into the world of Dimethylsulfoxide.

What Is DMSO?

Dimethylsulfoxide, commonly known as DMSO, is a powerful solvent and anti-inflammatory agent that has gained popularity in recent years for its potential health benefits. It was first discovered in the late 19th century by Russian scientist Alexander Zaytsev, but it wasn't until the 1960s that it started gaining attention for its unique properties.

In simple terms, DMSO is an organic compound with a chemical formula of $(CH_3)_2SO$. It is a colorless and odorless liquid at room temperature, with a slightly garlicky taste. However, when applied topically on the skin, it can have a strong sulfur-like smell due to the release of dimethyl sulfide.

DMSO is primarily derived from wood pulp and is commonly used as an industrial solvent in manufacturing processes. However, it has also been studied for its potential medical uses, particularly as a carrier agent for other substances due to its ability to easily penetrate biological membranes.

The exploration of Dimethyl sulfoxide (DMSO) in medical research has unveiled its potential as a valuable therapeutic agent for conditions like arthritis and interstitial cystitis. With promising initial findings, ongoing clinical trials aim to deepen our understanding of its efficacy and safety, paving the way for innovative treatments that could significantly improve patient outcomes. As research continues, DMSO may play a pivotal role in enhancing the quality of life for those suffering from chronic ailments.

Industrial Use

While medical researchers delved into the therapeutic benefits of DMSO, the chemical industry quickly recognized its unparalleled utility as a solvent. Its unique chemical properties allowed it to dissolve a wide array of compounds, making it an invaluable asset in multiple industrial applications.

- *Chemical Reactions:* In synthetic chemistry, DMSO served as a versatile solvent for diverse chemical reactions. Its ability to dissolve both organic and inorganic substances facilitated complex synthesis processes, enhancing reaction efficiency and yield.
- *Pharmaceutical Manufacturing*: The pharmaceutical industry leveraged DMSO's solvent capabilities for drug formulation and production. It was particularly useful in creating stable solutions for active pharmaceutical ingredients (APIs), ensuring the consistent potency and efficacy of medications.

- ***Cryoprotection***: Beyond its role as a solvent, DMSO became essential in the cryopreservation of biological materials. Its cryoprotective properties helped preserve cells, tissues, and organs at ultra-low temperatures, preventing ice crystal formation and cellular damage during freezing and thawing.
- ***Cleaning and Degreasing***: In the electronics and manufacturing sectors, DMSO was utilized for its powerful cleaning and degreasing properties. It efficiently removes contaminants from machinery and electronic components, preparing surfaces for subsequent processing or assembly.

The dual exploration of DMSO for medical and industrial purposes highlights its multifaceted applications. While clinical trials continue to unlock its therapeutic potential, its established role in the chemical and pharmaceutical industries underscores its versatility and indispensable value.

How Does DMSO Work?

Dimethyl sulfoxide (DMSO) is a highly versatile compound that exhibits a range of chemical and biological properties, making it useful in both medical and industrial applications. Understanding how DMSO works involves exploring its mechanisms of action, which include its ability to penetrate biological membranes, its anti-inflammatory and analgesic effects, and its role as a solvent.

1. **Penetration of Biological Membranes**

   DMSO is renowned for its exceptional ability to penetrate biological membranes, which is crucial for its effectiveness in various applications.

   - *Transdermal Carrier*: DMSO's small molecular size and polar nature allow it to easily traverse skin and other biological barriers. This property enables it to transport other compounds through the skin, enhancing the delivery of medications directly to target tissues.
   - *Cellular Permeability*: Once absorbed, DMSO increases the permeability of cell membranes, facilitating the entry of drugs and nutrients into cells and enhancing their therapeutic effects.

2. **Anti-inflammatory Properties**

   DMSO exhibits potent anti-inflammatory effects, which are central to its use in treating conditions such as arthritis and interstitial cystitis.

   - *Inhibition of Inflammatory Mediators*: DMSO reduces inflammation by inhibiting the production of pro-inflammatory cytokines and enzymes, such as prostaglandins and cyclooxygenase (COX). This decreases the inflammatory response and alleviates symptoms.

- ***Reduction of Oxidative Stress***: DMSO acts as a free radical scavenger, neutralizing reactive oxygen species (ROS) and reducing oxidative stress, which contributes to inflammation and tissue damage.

3. **Analgesic (Pain-Relieving) Effects**

The pain-relieving properties of DMSO make it valuable for managing chronic pain conditions.

- ***Blocking Pain Transmission***: DMSO interferes with nerve conduction fibers responsible for transmitting pain signals. This reduces the perception of pain at the application site.
- ***Alleviation of Muscle Spasms***: By modulating nerve activity, DMSO can also help relieve muscle spasms and cramps, providing further pain relief.

4. **Solvent Properties**

In industrial applications, DMSO's efficacy as a solvent is fundamental to its widespread use.

- ***Solubility***: DMSO's high polarity allows it to dissolve a wide range of organic and inorganic compounds, making it an effective solvent in pharmaceutical synthesis and other chemical processes.

- ***Cryoprotection***: In cryopreservation, DMSO prevents ice crystal formation, which can damage cellular structures. By stabilizing cells and tissues during freezing and thawing, DMSO ensures the viability of preserved biological samples.

5. **Cellular Protection and Recovery**

    DMSO aids in cellular protection and recovery, which is beneficial in both medical and laboratory settings.

    - ***Membrane Stabilization***: DMSO, or dimethyl sulfoxide, plays a crucial role in stabilizing cell membranes. By reinforcing their structure, it protects cells from damage that can be caused by external stressors such as harmful toxins, extreme temperatures, or mechanical injuries. This membrane stabilization is vital for maintaining cellular integrity and function, ensuring that cells remain resilient in challenging environments.
    - ***Enhanced Healing***: DMSO not only aids in membrane stabilization but also significantly enhances the healing process. By promoting improved blood circulation, it ensures that injured tissues receive the necessary nutrients and oxygen required for repair. Additionally, DMSO has anti-inflammatory properties that

help to reduce swelling and discomfort at the injury site. Together, these effects accelerate the healing process, allowing for quicker recovery and improved overall tissue health.

DMSO's multifaceted mechanisms of action—ranging from its membrane-penetrating ability and anti-inflammatory effects to its role as a solvent and cellular protector—make it a powerful tool in both medical and industrial contexts. Its unique properties enable it to deliver therapeutic benefits effectively while also serving diverse functional roles in various industries.

Different Types of DMSO

There are different types of DMSO available on the market, each with its specific uses and concentrations. Some commonly used types include:

1. **Pharmaceutical Grade**

   Pharmaceutical grade DMSO is the highest quality form available and is specifically intended for medical purposes. This grade adheres to strict purity standards set by regulatory bodies, ensuring that it is free from contaminants and suitable for human use.

   It is commonly prescribed by healthcare professionals for a variety of therapeutic applications, including the treatment of inflammatory conditions, pain management, and as a solvent for certain medications. Due to its high purity and stringent testing, pharmaceutical-grade DMSO is considered safe when used as directed by a medical professional.

2. **Industrial Grade**

   Industrial grade DMSO, on the other hand, does not meet the rigorous purity standards required for medical use. This type often contains impurities and additives that are not safe for human consumption or application. Its primary use is in industrial settings where high purity is not essential, such as in manufacturing processes, cleaning solvents, and paint strippers.

   While it is less expensive than pharmaceutical-grade DMSO, its potential contaminants make it unsuitable for therapeutic purposes. Using industrial-grade DMSO for medical reasons can pose significant health risks, including skin irritation, allergic reactions, or systemic toxicity.

3. **Gel or Cream**

   DMSO is also available in gel or cream formulations, which are designed for topical use and can be purchased over the counter. These products typically contain a lower concentration of DMSO, making them safer for general consumer use. They are commonly used for their analgesic properties, offering relief from muscle and joint pain, inflammation, and minor injuries.

The gel or cream form provides a convenient and easy-to-apply option, allowing users to target specific areas of discomfort without the need for a prescription. However, it is important to follow the manufacturer's instructions carefully to avoid potential side effects and ensure safe usage.

4. **Liquid**

The liquid form of DMSO is versatile and is often utilized in veterinary medicine. It can be administered orally, topically, or via injection, depending on the treatment requirements for animals. Veterinarians use liquid DMSO to manage pain, reduce inflammation, and treat various conditions in both large and small animals.

Its efficacy in penetrating tissues makes it a valuable tool in veterinary care. However, because of its potency and the need for precise dosing, the administration of liquid DMSO should always be overseen by a qualified veterinary professional to prevent adverse reactions and ensure the safety of the animal.

When using any type of DMSO, it is important to follow the recommended dosage and consult with a healthcare professional if you experience any adverse effects. Additionally, make sure to purchase from a reputable source and properly store the product according to its instructions. Incorrect use or storage can lead to contamination and potential harm.

Different Forms of DMSO and Their Uses

DMSO is available in various forms, each with its unique properties and usage. Some of the most common forms include:

1. **Topical Application**

    Topical application involves directly applying DMSO to the skin over the affected area. This method is widely used for its analgesic and anti-inflammatory properties, making it a popular choice for individuals seeking relief from conditions such as muscle strains, joint pain, and localized inflammation.

    The process typically involves using a gel, cream, or liquid form of DMSO, which is gently massaged onto the skin. Since DMSO has the unique ability to penetrate the skin and underlying tissues, it delivers therapeutic benefits directly to the site of discomfort. It is essential to ensure that the skin is clean and free from any other substances that could be carried into the body by DMSO's solvent properties. Users should also conduct a small patch test to check for any adverse reactions before proceeding with regular application.

2. **Injection**

    DMSO can also be administered via injection, a method most commonly performed in a medical setting under the supervision of a healthcare professional. This route of administration is typically reserved for more severe conditions that require rapid and concentrated delivery of DMSO's therapeutic effects.

    Conditions such as bladder infections (interstitial cystitis) and arthritis are examples where DMSO injections may be utilized. In these cases, DMSO is injected directly into the bladder or joints, respectively. The intravesical (bladder) application helps reduce inflammation and pain associated with chronic bladder conditions, while intra-articular injections can alleviate symptoms of arthritis. Given the invasive nature and potential risks of injections, it is crucial that this method is carried out by trained medical personnel to monitor for any complications and ensure proper dosing.

3. Oral Ingestion

Oral ingestion of DMSO, usually in liquid form, is another method of administration, though it is less common compared to topical application or injection. When taken orally, DMSO is absorbed through the gastrointestinal tract and distributed throughout the body, potentially providing systemic therapeutic effects.

This method may be considered for treating conditions that involve widespread inflammation or for individuals who prefer not to use topical or injectable forms. However, oral ingestion of DMSO can be associated with side effects such as gastrointestinal discomfort, garlic-like taste and breath odor, and dizziness.

Due to these potential side effects and the lack of standardized dosing guidelines, it is crucial to consult with a healthcare provider before using DMSO orally. The provider can offer guidance on appropriate dosing and monitor for any adverse reactions.

It is important to note that while DMSO can potentially provide relief for certain conditions, it is not a cure-all and should be used in conjunction with other treatments as recommended by a healthcare professional. It is also important to properly clean and disinfect any equipment used for DMSO administration to prevent contamination.

Use Cases of DMSO

DMSO (Dimethyl Sulfoxide) has been utilized for a multitude of conditions, each with differing levels of scientific backing. Here are some prevalent use cases:

1. **Pain Relief**

    DMSO is often used topically to alleviate pain, particularly in various conditions such as:

    - *Arthritis*: It can reduce joint pain and inflammation by penetrating deeply into the tissues. Many individuals with arthritis find significant relief from stiffness and discomfort with regular use.
    - *Tendinitis*: DMSO helps in decreasing swelling and enhancing mobility, making it easier for those suffering from tendinitis to continue their daily activities with less pain. It also promotes faster healing of the affected tendons.
    - *Muscle Injuries*: Athletes utilize it to expedite recovery from strains and sprains. By reducing muscle soreness and speeding up the healing

process, DMSO allows them to get back to their training routines more quickly. This makes it a popular choice among sports professionals and fitness enthusiasts.

2. **Inflammation Reduction**

   Its anti-inflammatory properties make DMSO useful in treating:

   - ***Interstitial Cystitis***: Applied directly to the bladder via a catheter, this treatment helps to reduce inflammation and alleviate pain, providing relief for those suffering from this chronic condition.
   - ***Skin Conditions***: Especially for conditions like scleroderma, which helps to soften hardened skin and reduce the appearance of lesions, thereby improving the overall skin texture and comfort for the patient.

3. **Wound Healing**

   DMSO promotes faster healing of wounds by:

   - Enhancing blood flow to the site.
   - Reducing tissue swelling and pain.
   - Preventing bacterial growth due to its antimicrobial properties.

4. **Ophthalmic Uses**

   It is used in eye drops for conditions like:

   - *Cataracts*: This condition involves the clouding of the eye's lens, leading to impaired vision. Certain treatments or preventive measures may help slow down or prevent the progression of cataracts, improving overall eye health and quality of life.
   - *Dry Eye Syndrome*: This common condition occurs when your eyes don't produce enough moisture or the right quality of tears, leading to discomfort and irritation. Various treatments can provide the necessary moisture and reduce irritation, helping to maintain eye comfort and function.

5. **Antioxidant Properties**

   As a potent free radical scavenger, DMSO is used in:

   - *Anti-aging treatments*: These treatments help to protect cells from oxidative damage, which can slow down the visible signs of aging and improve overall skin health.
   - *Cancer Therapy Support*: Some studies suggest that it might enhance the effectiveness of chemotherapy drugs, potentially improving

outcomes for patients undergoing cancer treatment.

6. **Drug Delivery Enhancement**

   DMSO is an excellent solvent and is thus used to:

   - Increase the absorption of other medications through the skin.
   - Act as a carrier to transport drugs more effectively into tissues.

7. **Neurological Benefits**

   Promising research suggests DMSO might aid in:

   - *Spinal Cord Injuries*: Research focuses on reducing the extent of damage caused by trauma to the spinal cord and promoting recovery through advanced therapies and interventions. Innovative treatments aim to restore mobility and improve the quality of life for affected individuals.
   - *Alzheimer's Disease*: Studies suggest that certain treatments might potentially slow down the progression of Alzheimer's disease due to their neuroprotective effects. By protecting brain cells from damage, these treatments could help preserve cognitive function and delay the onset of severe symptoms.

DMSO's versatility stems from its unique chemical properties, allowing it to penetrate biological membranes easily and exert wide-ranging therapeutic effects. While some uses are backed by substantial clinical evidence, others require further research to fully confirm their efficacy and safety.

Pros and Cons of DMSO

As with any medical treatment, there are both pros and cons to using DMSO. Here are some of the potential benefits and drawbacks to consider before using this compound.

Pros of Using DMSO

Dimethyl Sulfoxide (DMSO) offers several key advantages that make it a valuable substance in medical and pharmaceutical applications. Here are some of the primary advantages:

1. **Low Toxicity**

   Compared to many other solvents, DMSO has relatively low toxicity, especially when used in appropriate concentrations. This makes it safer for use in medical treatments and as a carrier for other drugs.

2. **Versatility**

   DMSO's versatility is one of its greatest strengths. It is used in a variety of fields, from medicine to veterinary practices, and even in industrial processes. Its broad range of applications makes it a valuable multi-purpose agent.

3. **Stability**

   DMSO is chemically stable under a wide range of conditions, which enhances its shelf life and makes it a reliable component in different formulations.

4. **Cryoprotectant**

   In biological research and medical procedures, DMSO is used as a cryoprotectant to preserve cells, tissues, and organs at very low temperatures. Its effectiveness in this role is critical for organ transplantation, fertility treatments, and biological research.

5. **Accessibility and Cost-Effectiveness**

   DMSO is relatively inexpensive and widely available, which makes it an accessible option for various treatments and applications. Its cost-effectiveness is particularly beneficial in settings with limited resources.

The advantages of using DMSO stem from its unique chemical properties, wide-ranging applications, and overall effectiveness. These characteristics make it a highly valuable tool in both medical and industrial contexts.

Cons

While DMSO has potential benefits, it is important to also consider the potential drawbacks of using this compound:

1. **Adverse Reactions**

    Some individuals may experience adverse reactions such as headaches, dizziness, and nausea. These symptoms are typically mild and manageable, especially when balanced against the significant pain relief and anti-inflammatory benefits that DMSO provides.

2. **Lack of Long-term Safety Data**

    While there is substantial evidence supporting the short-term benefits of DMSO, long-term safety data is limited. Ongoing research is needed to understand the potential risks associated with prolonged use. Nonetheless, the existing benefits for acute conditions make it a valuable treatment option.

3. **Interaction with Other Medications**

    Due to its property of enhancing drug absorption, DMSO can interact with other medications, potentially altering their efficacy or increasing the risk of side effects. Consulting a healthcare professional can mitigate these risks.

4. **Regulatory Restrictions**

   Despite its FDA approval for specific uses, DMSO is not universally approved for all conditions and is subject to regulatory restrictions in many countries. Adhering to local regulations and guidelines ensures its safe and legal use.

Despite these potential drawbacks, DMSO remains a widely used and beneficial therapy for various conditions. Its unique properties make it a valuable tool in managing pain and inflammation, especially in cases where conventional treatments have failed. As research continues, we can expect to gain a more comprehensive understanding of its benefits and limitations, leading to improved treatment options for individuals.

Potential Side Effects of DMSO

While DMSO has a relatively safe profile, it is not without potential side effects. These side effects are usually mild and do not occur in all individuals but should still be considered before using the therapy.

1. **Skin Irritation**

   DMSO can cause skin irritation when applied topically, leading to redness, itching, and burning sensation. To avoid this, it is recommended to test a small patch of skin before applying DMSO.

2. **Odor**

   DMSO has a strong garlic-like odor that may persist for several hours after application. This can be unpleasant for some individuals and may require taking precautions such as wearing a mask or applying the medication in a well-ventilated area.

3. **Burning Sensation**

   In some cases, DMSO can cause a burning sensation at the site of application. This is usually temporary and resolves on its own, but it may be uncomfortable for individuals.

4. **Nausea and Headaches**

   While rare, some individuals may experience nausea and headaches after using DMSO. These symptoms are usually mild and resolve quickly.

5. **Increase in Bleeding**

   DMSO has blood-thinning properties that can increase the risk of bleeding, especially when taken with other blood thinners such as aspirin or warfarin. Consulting a healthcare professional before using DMSO can help mitigate this risk.

6. **Allergic Reactions**

   Some individuals may be allergic to DMSO, leading to more severe reactions such as difficulty breathing and swelling of the face, tongue, or throat. In such cases, immediate medical attention should be sought.

These are just some of the potential side effects of using DMSO therapy. It is important to consult with a healthcare professional before beginning any new treatment and to carefully follow dosage instructions to minimize the risk of experiencing these side effects.

Potential Step-by-Step Guide To Get Started with DMSO

Using DMSO safely and effectively requires careful planning and consideration. The following step-by-step guide offers a structured approach to help you navigate the process. Remember, the importance of consulting with a healthcare professional cannot be overstated.

Step 1: Consultation

Seek Professional Advice

Before starting any treatment with DMSO, it is essential to consult with a healthcare provider who has experience and knowledge about its use. This initial step ensures that you are making an informed decision based on medical expertise, tailored to your specific health needs. Here's why this consultation is crucial:

Medical History Review

During the consultation, your healthcare provider will conduct a thorough review of your medical history. This comprehensive assessment typically includes:

- ***Overall Health***: It is important to discuss your general health status in detail, including any chronic illnesses or conditions that may have an impact on the safe and effective use of DMSO. This could encompass a range of health issues, from diabetes to respiratory conditions, and understanding your overall health can help your healthcare provider make better-informed decisions regarding your treatment.
- ***Current Medications***: Please provide a comprehensive and detailed list of all medications you are currently taking, including prescription drugs, supplements, herbal remedies, and over-the-counter medications. This information is crucial for your healthcare provider to identify any potential interactions between DMSO and these substances, ensuring your safety and the effectiveness of your treatment plan.
- ***Pre-existing Conditions***: It's essential to share any known medical conditions you may have, such as liver or kidney disease, cardiovascular issues, skin disorders, or allergies. Certain pre-existing conditions can lead to contraindications for the use of DMSO or may require specific precautions to be taken to ensure

your health and safety during treatment. Being thorough in your disclosure can lead to a more tailored and effective healthcare strategy.

Allergy Check

An essential part of the consultation involves evaluating your allergy history to ensure you are not allergic to DMSO or related compounds. This step includes:

- *Allergy History*: It is crucial to discuss any known allergies with your healthcare provider, particularly those related to sulfur-containing compounds. Since DMSO (dimethyl sulfoxide) is an organosulfur compound, understanding your allergy history can help prevent potentially dangerous reactions and ensure safe use. This includes being aware of any past allergic reactions you have experienced, as well as the severity and nature of those reactions.
- *Skin Sensitivity*: If you have sensitive skin or a history of dermatitis, it is essential to communicate this to your healthcare provider. They may recommend conducting a patch test, which involves applying a small amount of DMSO to a discreet patch of skin. This test can help identify any adverse reactions or sensitivities you may have before you commit to using DMSO more broadly on your skin. This precaution is particularly important for individuals with a history of

skin issues, as it helps ensure that the treatment is safe and suitable for your specific skin type.

- ***Previous Reactions***: Always inform your healthcare provider about any previous adverse reactions you have experienced with topical treatments or solvents. This information can significantly influence your suitability for DMSO use. If you've had negative reactions to similar compounds in the past, your provider may want to take extra precautions or consider alternative treatments that may be safer for you. Understanding your medical history in this context is vital for optimizing your treatment plan and minimizing risks.

Dosage Recommendations

Based on the information gathered during the consultation, your healthcare provider will offer personalized dosage recommendations. These recommendations are critical to ensuring the safe and effective use of DMSO.

Key considerations include:

- ***Condition-Specific Dosage***: The appropriate concentration and dosage of DMSO vary depending on the condition being treated. For instance, lower concentrations may be advised for sensitive skin areas, while higher concentrations might be suitable for more severe conditions.

- ***Frequency of Application***: Your provider will suggest how often you should apply DMSO. The frequency can range from daily applications to more spaced-out intervals, depending on your treatment plan and skin tolerance.
- ***Duration of Treatment***: Discuss the expected duration of DMSO use. Long-term use may require periodic evaluations to monitor effectiveness and safety, while short-term use might necessitate follow-up consultations to assess outcomes.

Additional Considerations

In addition to the core aspects of the consultation, your healthcare provider might address other relevant factors:

1. **Lifestyle and Habits**

   Certain lifestyle factors, such as smoking, alcohol consumption, and diet, can significantly impact both the effectiveness and safety of DMSO treatment. For instance, smoking can reduce circulation and hinder healing processes, while excessive alcohol can interfere with liver function and drug metabolism.

   Your healthcare provider may offer tailored advice on lifestyle adjustments, such as adopting a balanced diet rich in antioxidants and staying hydrated, to enhance treatment outcomes and promote overall well-being.

2. **Concurrent Therapies**

   If you are undergoing other treatments or therapies, such as physical therapy, acupuncture, or herbal medicine, it is crucial to discuss these with your healthcare provider. Each therapy has its unique mechanisms and potential interactions.

   Understanding the full scope of your treatment regimen helps ensure that DMSO is integrated safely and effectively without compromising the benefits of your other therapies. This thorough communication allows for more personalized care and better health outcomes.

3. **Monitoring Plan**

   Establishing a detailed plan for monitoring your progress and any side effects is vital to the success of your treatment. Regular check-ins with your healthcare provider can help track the effectiveness of DMSO and identify any adverse reactions early on.

   This may include scheduled appointments to assess pain levels, mobility, and overall health, as well as any necessary adjustments to your treatment plan based on your response to DMSO. Keeping a journal of your symptoms and any changes can also be a helpful tool in this monitoring process, ensuring that you receive optimal care throughout your treatment journey.

By engaging in a comprehensive consultation with a knowledgeable healthcare provider, you lay the foundation for a safe and informed approach to using DMSO. This initial step is vital for tailoring the treatment to your individual needs, minimizing risks, and optimizing therapeutic benefits.

Step 2: Choosing the Right Concentration

Understanding Concentrations

DMSO (Dimethyl sulfoxide) is a versatile compound available in various concentrations, each suited for different applications and conditions. Choosing the right concentration is crucial for ensuring both efficacy and safety.

Range of Concentrations

DMSO solutions typically range from 10% to 90%, with each concentration offering different benefits and risks:

1. ***Lower Concentrations (10%-30%)***: These are generally used for sensitive areas such as the face or mucous membranes and for individuals new to DMSO. Lower concentrations reduce the risk of skin irritation and other side effects, making them a safer starting point for most users. They are also suitable for delicate skin types or when applying DMSO near sensitive tissues.

    Example Use Cases:

- Mild arthritis symptoms in hands and feet.
- Initial treatment phases to assess tolerance.
- Topical application on sensitive skin areas.

2. ***Medium Concentrations (30%-70%)***: These concentrations are commonly used for moderate conditions and general applications. Medium concentrations strike a balance between effectiveness and safety, providing more potent anti-inflammatory and analgesic effects while minimizing severe reactions.

Example Use Cases:

- Moderate to severe arthritis in larger joints like knees and shoulders.
- Muscular aches and pains.
- General anti-inflammatory applications for recurring conditions.

3. ***Higher Concentrations (70%-90%)***: Reserved for more severe conditions and should be used under professional supervision. Higher concentrations can offer significant relief for intense pain and inflammation but carry a higher risk of skin irritation, blistering, and other adverse reactions.

Example Use Cases:

- Severe and chronic inflammatory conditions.

- Interstitial cystitis treatments under clinical guidance.
- Situations requiring deep tissue penetration for therapeutic effects.

Dilution Guidelines

If you need to adjust the concentration of your DMSO solution, proper dilution is essential. Improper dilution can lead to ineffective treatment or increase the risk of adverse reactions.

Steps for Safe Dilution

1. *Use Distilled Water*: Always use distilled water for diluting DMSO. Tap water or regular bottled water may contain impurities that could interact with DMSO and cause irritation or reduce its effectiveness.
2. *Calculate Desired Concentration*: Determine the final concentration you need. For instance, if you want to dilute a 90% DMSO solution to 30%, you would need to mix one part of the 90% solution with two parts distilled water.
    - *Calculation Example*: To make 100 mL of 30% DMSO from 90%, you would mix approximately 33.3 mL of 90% DMSO with 66.7 mL of distilled water.
3. *Mix Thoroughly*: Combine the DMSO and distilled water in a clean glass or plastic container. Mix

thoroughly to ensure an even concentration throughout the solution.
4. ***Store Properly***: Store the diluted solution in a tightly sealed container, away from direct sunlight and extreme temperatures. Label the container with the concentration and date of preparation.

Handling Precautions

- ***Wear Protective Gear***: Always wear gloves when handling DMSO to avoid skin contact, as it rapidly penetrates the skin and can carry other substances with it.
- ***Clean Mixing Tools***: Ensure all mixing containers and tools are clean and free from contaminants. Any impurities can be carried into the body through the DMSO application.
- ***Test Before Use***: After dilution, perform a patch test to check for any adverse reactions before applying the solution to larger areas.

Practical Tips for Application

- ***Start Low***: If you are new to DMSO, start with a lower concentration and gradually increase it based on your tolerance and the advice of your healthcare provider.
- ***Observe Reactions***: Carefully monitor the treated area for any signs of irritation, redness, or discomfort.

Adjust the concentration accordingly if adverse reactions occur.
- **Consult Healthcare Providers**: Always follow the guidance of healthcare professionals regarding the appropriate concentration and application frequency tailored to your condition.

By understanding the appropriate concentrations and following safe dilution practices, you can maximize the benefits of DMSO while minimizing the risk of side effects. This careful approach ensures a safer and more effective treatment experience.

Step 3: Preparation

Gathering Supplies

Preparation is key to ensuring a safe and effective application of DMSO. Before you begin, it's important to gather all necessary supplies to avoid interruptions during the process. Here's a detailed list of what you'll need and why each item is essential:

1. ***DMSO Solution (at the recommended concentration):*** The specific concentration recommended by your healthcare provider is crucial for targeting your condition effectively while minimizing potential side effects. Ensure that the solution matches the concentration advised.

2. ***Distilled Water (for dilution, if needed)***: If you need to adjust the concentration of your DMSO, distilled water is required for safe dilution. Unlike tap water, distilled water is free from impurities that could cause irritation or reduce the effectiveness of the DMSO.
3. ***Clean Glass or Plastic Container for Mixing***: A clean container is necessary for mixing DMSO with distilled water if dilution is needed. Avoid metal containers as they can react with DMSO. Glass or plastic is preferred for maintaining the purity of the solution.
4. ***Disposable Gloves***: DMSO can rapidly penetrate the skin and carry other substances with it, potentially causing unwanted side effects. Wearing disposable gloves prevents direct contact with the DMSO, ensuring safety during application.
5. ***Cotton Balls or Applicator Pads***: These are used to apply the DMSO solution to the skin. Cotton balls and applicator pads provide an even and controlled application, helping to avoid over-saturation of the area being treated.
6. ***Mild Soap and Water***: Cleaning the application area with mild soap and water removes dirt, oils, and any other contaminants from the skin. This step ensures better absorption of the DMSO and reduces the risk of irritation.

Conducting a Patch Test

Before applying DMSO extensively, it is crucial to conduct a patch test. This test helps determine whether you have any allergic reactions or skin sensitivity to the solution. Follow these steps for a thorough patch test:

1. *Apply a Small Amount of Diluted DMSO to a Patch of Skin*
    - *Location*: Select a small, discreet area on your forearm for application. The forearm is particularly ideal for this purpose as it is easily accessible for both application and monitoring. Additionally, this area allows for clear observation of the skin's response, making it simpler to detect any potential reactions or sensitivities.
    - *Method*: Using a cotton ball or applicator pad, carefully apply a small amount of the diluted DMSO solution to the chosen patch of skin. It's important to use gentle pressure while applying to ensure that the solution is evenly distributed across the area. This will help maximize the effectiveness of the treatment while minimizing any discomfort. After application, monitor the area closely for any changes or reactions over time.

2. **Wait 24 Hours**
   - ***Observation Period***: Allow the DMSO to remain on your skin for a full 24 hours without washing it off. This duration is crucial, as it provides ample time to monitor any potential delayed reactions that may occur, such as redness, irritation, or allergic responses. Keeping track of how your skin reacts during this time can offer valuable insights into your sensitivity to the substance.
   - ***Protect the Area***: It is important to avoid covering the test area with clothing, bandages, or any other materials that could interfere with the observation process. Keeping the area exposed to air not only allows for better ventilation but also helps you notice any immediate or subtle changes more easily. This approach enhances the accuracy of your observations and ensures that the test is conducted effectively.

3. **Observe for Signs of Irritation, Redness, or Discomfort**
   - ***Immediate Reactions***: Within the first few hours after exposure, it's important to carefully check for any signs of redness, itching, burning, or swelling in the test area. These symptoms can indicate an allergic reaction or heightened

skin sensitivity, which may require prompt attention. If any of these issues arise, consider removing the substance and consulting with a healthcare professional for further guidance.

- *Delayed Reactions*: After the initial period, continue to monitor the test area closely throughout the entire 24-hour period for any delayed responses. Some allergic reactions or sensitivities may take longer to manifest, and it's crucial to remain vigilant during this time. Keep an eye out for changes in skin texture, additional irritation, or the development of blisters, as these could signify a more serious reaction that warrants immediate medical evaluation.

4. **Proceed Based on Results**

    - *No Adverse Reactions*: If no signs of irritation, redness, or discomfort are observed after 24 hours, it is generally safe to proceed with the full application of DMSO. However, continue to follow the guidance of your healthcare provider regarding the application process.
    - *Adverse Reactions*: If you experience any adverse reactions during the patch test, do not proceed with the full application. Contact your healthcare provider immediately for further advice. They may recommend a lower

concentration, alternative application method, or discontinuation of use.

Additional Tips for Preparation

- *Environment*: Choose a clean, well-ventilated area for preparing and applying DMSO. Good ventilation helps dissipate any odors and ensures a comfortable environment.
- *Labeling*: Clearly label your DMSO solutions, especially if you are using multiple concentrations. Include the concentration and date of preparation to avoid any confusion.
- *Hygiene*: Maintain strict hygiene throughout the preparation process. Ensure all tools and containers are sanitized to prevent contamination.

By thoroughly preparing and conducting a patch test, you can significantly reduce the risk of adverse reactions and ensure a smoother and more effective treatment experience.

Step 4: Application Method

Applying DMSO correctly is crucial to maximize its therapeutic benefits while minimizing potential side effects. The following expanded guide provides detailed instructions for each part of the application process.

Clean the Application Area

Before applying DMSO, it's vital to clean the area where you intend to apply the solution. Proper cleaning ensures better absorption and reduces the risk of irritation or contamination.

1. ***Select the Area***: Begin by carefully identifying the specific area on your body that requires treatment. This could be joints affected by arthritis, muscles experiencing soreness or tension, or any other inflamed regions that cause discomfort. Taking the time to pinpoint the exact area of concern will help ensure that you focus on what needs the most attention.

2. ***Use Mild Soap***: Opt for a mild, fragrance-free soap specifically designed for sensitive skin to avoid introducing additional irritants. Harsh soaps can strip the skin of its natural oils, leading to dryness or causing allergic reactions. Such reactions can potentially interfere with the effectiveness of DMSO (Dimethyl Sulfoxide) by affecting how well it penetrates the skin.

3. ***Wash Thoroughly***: Begin by wetting the area with lukewarm water. Next, apply the mild soap generously across the skin. Gently rub the skin in circular motions to effectively remove dirt, oils, and any other substances that may have accumulated. Pay special attention to areas that may have accumulated sweat,

dead skin cells, or environmental pollutants, as these can hinder both cleanliness and the efficacy of subsequent treatments.

4. **Rinse Completely**: It's crucial to ensure that all soap is thoroughly rinsed off with clean, lukewarm water. Any soap residue left on the skin can interact negatively with DMSO, hindering its absorption and potentially causing irritation. Take your time with this step to ensure no traces of soap remain.

5. **Dry the Area**: Gently pat the area dry with a clean, soft towel. It's important to avoid rubbing the skin too harshly, as this can lead to irritation or discomfort. Make sure the skin is completely dry before proceeding with the application of DMSO, as moisture can also affect its absorption and overall effectiveness. Proper preparation of the skin sets the stage for optimal results.

Applying DMSO

Proper application technique is essential for ensuring the safety and effectiveness of DMSO.

1. **Wear Gloves**
   - **Importance**: DMSO can penetrate the skin quickly and carry other substances along with it, potentially causing unwanted effects. Wearing disposable gloves (preferably nitrile or latex)

prevents direct contact with the solution and protects your skin from unintended exposure.
- *Procedure*: Put on a pair of disposable gloves before handling the DMSO solution. Ensure the gloves are clean and free from any residues.

2. *Use an Applicator*
   - *Choosing an Applicator*: Select a clean cotton ball, applicator pad, or gauze for applying the DMSO. These materials provide a controlled and even distribution of the solution.
   - *Soaking the Applicator*: Pour a small amount of the DMSO solution into a clean container. Dip the cotton ball, applicator pad, or gauze into the solution until it is adequately soaked but not dripping.

3. *Apply Evenly*
   - *Application Technique*: Gently apply the soaked applicator to the affected area. Use light, even strokes to cover the entire surface evenly. Avoid vigorous rubbing or massaging, as this can cause irritation or drive DMSO deeper into the skin than intended.
   - *Coverage*: Ensure that the application covers the entire targeted area uniformly. Over-saturating one spot can lead to irritation,

while insufficient coverage may reduce the effectiveness of the treatment.

4. *Allow to Dry*
    - *Drying Time*: Let the DMSO solution dry naturally on the skin. Typically, this process takes about 15-20 minutes. During this time, avoid touching or disturbing the treated area to allow for optimal absorption.
    - *Avoid Covering*: Do not cover the applied area with clothing or any other material until the DMSO has fully dried. Covering the area prematurely can trap moisture and impede the drying process, potentially leading to irritation or reduced efficacy.
    - *Ventilation*: If possible, apply DMSO in a well-ventilated area to help dissipate any odors and facilitate drying. Good airflow can make the application process more comfortable and effective.

Additional Tips for Application

- **Consistency**: It is crucial to apply DMSO at the same time each day to maintain consistent therapeutic levels in your system. This regularity helps optimize its effectiveness, allowing your body to adapt and respond to the treatment more efficiently over time.

- **Skin Care**: Once DMSO has dried completely, you can apply a gentle moisturizer to the treated area. This step is important for preventing dryness and ensuring the health of your skin. Choose a moisturizer that is free from fragrances and other potential irritants, as these can compromise the integrity of the skin barrier and lead to irritation.
- **Avoid Contaminants**: To ensure the best absorption and efficacy of DMSO, keep the application area clean and free from contaminants throughout the drying process. Even small particles like dust, pet hair, and other debris can adhere to the wet DMSO, potentially being carried into the skin and causing unwanted reactions. Taking the time to prepare a clean environment for application will enhance the overall effectiveness of the treatment.

By following these detailed steps for cleaning and applying DMSO, you can enhance the treatment's effectiveness while minimizing the risk of adverse reactions. Consistent and careful application ensures that you derive the maximum benefits from using DMSO.

Step 5: Monitoring and Adjusting

Observation

Monitoring the treated area after applying DMSO is crucial to ensure safety and effectiveness. This step involves keen observation of both immediate and delayed reactions, as well as keeping detailed records of your observations.

Immediate Reactions

After applying DMSO, pay close attention to the treated area for any immediate signs of irritation or adverse reactions. These reactions typically manifest within the first few hours and may include:

- ***Redness***: Pay close attention to any unusual redness around the application site. While mild redness is often a normal response to topical treatments, a significant increase in redness could indicate irritation or an allergic reaction. If you notice this, it's advisable to stop using the product and consult with a healthcare professional.
- ***Itching***: Be vigilant for any itching sensations that may arise soon after application. This itching can vary in intensity, from mild discomfort to severe irritation, and should be carefully noted. Persistent itching could suggest a sensitivity to the product or an allergic reaction, warranting further investigation.
- ***Burning***: Keep an eye out for any burning sensations occurring on the skin after applying the treatment. This discomfort may signal an adverse reaction to the concentration or formulation of DMSO being used. If the burning sensation is intense or lasts for an extended

period, it is critical to wash off the product and seek medical advice.

- ***Swelling***: Regularly check for any swelling in the treated area. Swelling can indicate an allergic reaction or irritation and should be taken seriously. If you observe swelling that persists or worsens, it's important to discontinue use and reach out to a healthcare provider for guidance and evaluation.

Delayed Reactions

In addition to immediate responses, it's important to observe the treated area over the next 24-48 hours. Delayed reactions can provide further insight into your skin's tolerance and the suitability of the treatment:

- ***Increased Sensitivity***: Pay close attention to whether there is a heightened sensitivity in the treated area. This could manifest as tenderness, discomfort, or an unusual response to touch, which may indicate that your skin is reacting to the treatment. It's important to monitor how this sensitivity evolves over time, as it can guide you in assessing your skin's condition and the effectiveness of the treatment.
- ***Prolonged Discomfort***: Keep an eye out for any ongoing discomfort that lingers beyond the initial application period. This may include prolonged itching, burning sensations, or persistent pain that doesn't subside. If these symptoms continue, it's

advisable to evaluate the treatment and consider consulting a healthcare professional, as they could signify an adverse reaction or sensitivity to the product used.

- ***Skin Changes***: Be vigilant for any alterations in skin texture or appearance following the treatment. Look for signs such as dryness, excessive peeling, or blister formation, which could indicate an adverse reaction. Noting these changes is crucial, as they can provide insights into how your skin is responding and whether you should adjust your skincare routine or seek professional advice.

Record-Keeping

Maintain a journal to document your observations. Include details such as:

- Date and time of application.
- Concentration of DMSO used.
- Specific area treated.
- Immediate and delayed reactions were observed.
- Any additional notes or relevant symptoms.

This record will be valuable for both self-monitoring and discussions with your healthcare provider.

Adjusting Treatment

Based on your observations, you may need to adjust your treatment plan to optimize safety and effectiveness. Here are some common adjustments:

1. *Reduce Concentration*

   If you experience significant irritation or adverse reactions, consider using a lower concentration of DMSO:

   - *Dilution*: To achieve a lower concentration of the DMSO solution, carefully dilute the current solution with distilled water. It is important to follow the specific dilution guidelines outlined in Step 2 to ensure accuracy and effectiveness in the resulting mixture. This step is crucial, as the right dilution can enhance the safety and efficacy of the application.
   - *Re-evaluation*: After preparing the new concentration, conduct another patch test on a small area of skin to assess its tolerance and ensure it does not cause any adverse reactions. This step is vital, as skin sensitivities can vary, and confirming that the diluted solution is well-tolerated will help prevent any potential irritation when applied to larger areas.

- ***Professional Guidance***: Always consult your healthcare provider for personalized advice on the appropriate concentration of DMSO for your specific condition. They can offer valuable insights based on your individual health needs and circumstances, ensuring that you use the solution safely and effectively. Their expertise can guide you in making informed decisions about your treatment plan.

2. **Modify Frequency**

Adjust the frequency of application based on your skin's response and the guidance of your healthcare provider:

- ***Decrease Frequency***: If you experience any signs of irritation or discomfort, it's important to reduce the frequency of application. For instance, if you were using DMSO on a daily basis, consider adjusting your routine to apply it every other day. This allows your skin to recover and minimizes the risk of adverse reactions while still benefiting from the treatment.
- ***Increase Frequency***: On the other hand, if you find that the treatment is well-tolerated and your healthcare provider recommends it, you might think about gradually increasing the frequency

of application. This could help you achieve more effective therapeutic results over time, as your body may adapt to the treatment and better respond to its effects. Always consult with your healthcare provider before making adjustments.

- *Consistency*: It's crucial to maintain a consistent application schedule. Keeping your routine steady helps you monitor how any changes in frequency impact your condition. By recording your experiences, you can provide valuable insights to your healthcare provider, allowing for more tailored adjustments to your treatment plan. Consistency not only aids in tracking progress but also helps to establish a routine that your body can rely on for optimal results.

3. *Discontinue Use*

If severe reactions occur, it is crucial to stop using DMSO immediately and seek medical advice:

- *Severe Symptoms*: If you experience signs such as an intense burning sensation, significant swelling in the affected area, blistering, or severe discomfort that impacts your daily activities, it is crucial to immediately discontinue the use of DMSO. These symptoms may indicate a serious reaction, and continuing use could potentially lead to further complications.

- ***Medical Consultation***: It is essential to contact your healthcare provider as soon as possible to discuss these reactions in detail. They can assess your symptoms and explore alternative treatment options tailored to your specific needs. Depending on your situation, they may recommend different concentrations of DMSO, alternative formulations that are gentler on the skin, or entirely different therapies that may be more suitable for your condition. Always prioritize your health and well-being by seeking professional guidance.

4. **Long-term Monitoring**

Continue to monitor your condition and the treated area over the long term, even if initial reactions are mild. Regular check-ins with your healthcare provider can help ensure the continued safety and effectiveness of the treatment:

- ***Periodic Evaluations***: It's essential to schedule regular follow-up appointments with your healthcare provider to closely assess your progress. These evaluations will allow for a comprehensive review of how you are responding to the treatment, enabling your provider to identify any areas that may need adjustment. By actively engaging in these discussions, you can ensure that your treatment plan remains aligned with your health goals and any changes in your condition.

- *Holistic Approach*: In addition to DMSO treatment, consider incorporating other supportive therapies and lifestyle modifications that can enhance its overall effectiveness. This might include nutritional counseling, physical therapy, or mindfulness practices such as yoga and meditation. By taking a holistic approach, you can optimize your well-being and support your body in achieving the best possible outcomes from your treatment.

By diligently observing and adjusting your treatment based on your skin's reactions and professional advice, you can tailor the use of DMSO to your specific needs, ensuring both safety and optimal therapeutic outcomes.

Step 6: Long-term Considerations

1. **Consistent Monitoring**

    Long-term use of DMSO necessitates ongoing and consistent monitoring to ensure the treatment remains safe and effective over time. This involves maintaining detailed records of your dosage, the frequency of application, and any observed effects, both positive and negative. It is also crucial to stay vigilant for any changes in your overall condition or health status, as these may indicate the need for adjustments in your treatment plan.

Regular check-ins with a healthcare professional can provide valuable insights and help address any concerns that may arise during your use of DMSO. This proactive approach can enhance the safety and efficacy of the treatment, ensuring you achieve the best possible outcomes.

2. Keep a Journal

Maintaining a journal is an essential part of long-term monitoring. Your journal should include:

- *Application Times and Dates*: It's important to meticulously record every instance of DMSO application by noting the exact dates and times. Keeping a detailed log helps you track the frequency and consistency of your treatment, allowing you to analyze patterns over time and make informed adjustments as needed.
- *Concentration Levels Used*: Be sure to document the concentration of DMSO applied during each session. This information is crucial for identifying any correlation between different

concentration levels and the occurrence of side effects or therapeutic outcomes. Understanding how varying concentrations affect your treatment can lead to more effective use of DMSO.

- ***Observed Effects or Side Effects***: Take careful note of any immediate or delayed reactions you experience, as well as any improvements or worsening of your symptoms. Include comprehensive details such as instances of redness, itching, pain relief, or the emergence of new symptoms. This thorough documentation will provide valuable insights into your overall response to the treatment and help guide future decisions.

3. Periodic Self-Assessment

In addition to professional evaluations, regularly assess your own health and condition. Pay attention to:

- ***Symptom Changes***: It's important to closely monitor any variations in the symptoms for which you are using DMSO. Take detailed notes on any improvements you experience, such as reduced pain or inflammation, as well as any deteriorations, like increased discomfort or new symptoms that may arise. Keeping a symptom diary can help you track these changes over time.

- **Skin Condition**: Pay careful attention to any changes in the skin where DMSO is applied. This includes not only dryness or irritation but also any signs of redness, swelling, or rashes. If you notice persistent issues, consider consulting a healthcare professional to ensure that the application is safe and suitable for your skin type.
- **General Health**: It's crucial to maintain an awareness of your overall well-being while using DMSO. Regularly assess your energy levels and mood, and take note of any new symptoms that develop over time, such as fatigue, headaches, or changes in appetite. Engaging in self-reflection and possibly discussing these observations with a healthcare provider can enhance your understanding of how DMSO affects your health in the long run.

4. **Periodic Evaluations**

Regular check-ins with your healthcare provider are crucial for the ongoing assessment of DMSO's effectiveness and safety. These evaluations can help determine whether to continue, adjust, or discontinue your treatment.

5. **Schedule Regular Appointments**
    - *Frequency*: Depending on your specific condition and tailored treatment plan, it is crucial to schedule evaluations at regular intervals. These could be monthly, bi-monthly, or quarterly, allowing for consistent monitoring of your progress and timely adjustments to your care.
    - *Comprehensive Review*: During these appointments, your healthcare provider will conduct a thorough review of your journal, which should detail your experiences, symptoms, and any changes you've noticed. This discussion will encompass any observed effects of the treatment, and your provider may also perform necessary physical exams or diagnostic tests to gather more information and assess your overall health.
    - *Adjustments*: Based on the findings from your evaluations and discussions, your healthcare provider may recommend specific adjustments to your treatment plan. This could include changes to the concentration of your medication, modifications to the frequency of application, or the introduction of additional treatments to enhance overall effectiveness and minimize potential side effects, ensuring you

receive the best possible care tailored to your needs.

6. **Professional Guidance**
    - *Expert Advice*: Regular consultations with your healthcare provider are crucial for ensuring that you receive expert guidance tailored to your specific needs and circumstances. These sessions provide an opportunity to discuss any concerns, monitor your progress, and adjust your treatment plan as necessary, all while fostering a trusting relationship that enhances your overall healthcare experience.
    - *Emerging Research*: Staying informed about new research and developments related to DMSO is vital for making informed decisions about your treatment. Engaging in discussions with your healthcare provider allows you to gain valuable insights and updates on the latest findings, potential benefits, and risks associated with DMSO. This knowledge can significantly enhance your treatment plan and empower you to make choices that align with your health goals.

7. **Long-term Safety**

    Awareness of the long-term implications of using DMSO is vital for maintaining health and preventing complications. While DMSO can be beneficial, prolonged use requires careful management.

8. **Skin Health**

Continual application of DMSO can lead to skin-related issues, so it's important to manage and mitigate these risks:

- *Dryness and Irritation*: Regular use of DMSO can lead to dryness or irritation of the skin due to its solvent properties. To prevent this discomfort, it's advisable to take breaks from the DMSO application as recommended by your healthcare provider. In addition, using moisturizing creams or lotions that are free from fragrances and irritants can be beneficial. Look for products that contain soothing ingredients, such as aloe vera or shea butter, which can help hydrate and protect the skin while alleviating any potential irritation.
- *Monitoring for Reactions*: It is crucial to continuously monitor the treated areas for any signs of worsening irritation, such as increased redness, swelling, or the development of new skin issues. Being vigilant about these changes can help ensure that any adverse reactions are addressed promptly. If you notice any concerning symptoms or changes in your skin

condition, make sure to report these to your healthcare provider as soon as possible to receive appropriate guidance and care. Your health and comfort should always be a priority.

9. **Overall Well-being**

Regularly assess your general health and report any unusual symptoms to your healthcare provider:

- *Systemic Effects*: While DMSO is mainly used topically for its anti-inflammatory and pain-relieving benefits, it can still produce systemic effects that impact the entire body. Watch for symptoms like headaches, dizziness, nausea, or other unusual reactions after application. These reactions can vary in intensity based on individual sensitivity and dosage, so monitoring your body's response is essential.
- *Holistic Health*: When assessing DMSO's effects, consider it in the context of your overall health. This includes not only its topical use but also its interaction with your diet, exercise, stress levels, and other medications. A holistic approach supports your body in various ways, leading to better health and a clearer understanding of DMSO's role in your wellness strategy. It may be helpful to consult a

healthcare provider to discuss how DMSO and other factors can work together for your benefit.

Using DMSO can be a valuable tool for managing certain conditions when applied correctly and safely. This chapter has provided a comprehensive step-by-step guide to help you navigate the application process. Remember, the key to successful and safe use of DMSO lies in informed decision-making, professional consultation, and diligent monitoring.

Best Practices for Maximizing Benefits and Minimizing Risks

While DMSO has shown potential therapeutic benefits, it is important to use the product responsibly and with caution. Here are some best practices for maximizing benefits and minimizing risks:

1. ***Follow Dosage Recommendations***: Always adhere to recommended dosages and dilution ratios when using DMSO to avoid potential side effects and toxicity. It's important to follow the guidelines provided by your healthcare provider or the product instructions carefully.
2. ***Regular Monitoring***: Regularly monitor for any side effects, such as skin irritation or unusual symptoms. If you notice anything unusual, consult your healthcare

provider immediately. Keeping track of how you feel can help in adjusting the treatment as needed.

3. ***Storage***: Store DMSO in a cool, dry place to maintain its effectiveness and prevent degradation. Proper storage is crucial to ensure the product remains safe and effective for use. Avoid exposing it to direct sunlight or extreme temperatures.

4. ***Combine with Other Therapies***: DMSO can be more effective when used as part of a broader treatment plan, especially for conditions like osteoarthritis, muscle pain, and inflammation. Discuss with your healthcare provider the possibility of combining DMSO with other therapies or medications to enhance its benefits.

5. ***Hydration***: Stay well-hydrated while using DMSO, as it can cause dehydration when used extensively. Drinking plenty of water is essential to help your body process and eliminate the compound efficiently, reducing the risk of dehydration and related complications.

Following these best practices can help you get the most out of DMSO while ensuring your safety and well-being. Additionally, it's essential to consult with your healthcare provider before incorporating DMSO into your treatment plan, especially if you have pre-existing medical conditions or are taking other medications. They can provide personalized recommendations and monitor your progress to ensure optimal results.

Moreover, it's crucial to note that DMSO is not a cure-all and should not be relied upon as the sole treatment for any condition. It works differently for each individual, and its effects may vary depending on the underlying cause. Therefore, it's vital to use DMSO responsibly as part of a comprehensive treatment plan prescribed by a healthcare professional.

Safety Precautions and Consideration for DMSO Usage

DMSO is a powerful and versatile therapeutic agent, but it is not without its risks and limitations. In this chapter, we will delve deeper into the safety precautions and considerations that should be taken when using DMSO as part of your treatment plan.

Dosage Instructions

As mentioned in previous chapters, following the prescribed dosage instructions for DMSO is crucial for achieving optimal therapeutic outcomes. It is important to note that dosing may differ depending on the condition being treated and individual patient needs. Therefore, always follow the specific dosing instructions provided by your healthcare provider or those found on the product label.

Skipping doses or deviating from the recommended dosage can disrupt the effectiveness of the treatment and increase the risk of adverse effects. In some cases, it may even result in serious health complications.

Adverse Effects

DMSO is generally well-tolerated by most individuals; however, like any medication or therapy, it may cause adverse effects in some people. These can range from mild discomfort to severe reactions. Some of the commonly reported side effects associated with DMSO usage include:

- Skin irritation or burning sensation at the application site
- Unpleasant taste and odor (when used orally)
- Nausea and vomiting
- Headache
- Dizziness
- Diarrhea

If you experience any of these symptoms, it is important to inform your healthcare provider immediately. They may advise you to discontinue DMSO usage or adjust the dosage to alleviate the adverse effects.

Precautions and Warnings

While DMSO is generally considered safe, certain precautions and warnings must be taken into consideration when using this therapeutic agent.

1. **Allergic Reactions**

    Individuals who are hypersensitive to DMSO should not use this medication. In some cases, severe allergic reactions can occur, which may require immediate medical attention. If you experience symptoms such as difficulty breathing, wheezing, or swelling of the face or throat, seek medical help right away.

2. **Use in Pregnant and Breastfeeding Women**

   There is limited information on the safety of DMSO usage during pregnancy and breastfeeding. Therefore, it is recommended to consult with your healthcare provider before using this medication in these situations.

3. **Interactions with Other Medications**

   DMSO may interact with certain medications, including blood thinners, steroids, and some antibiotics. It is important to inform your doctor about all the medications you are currently taking before starting DMSO treatment.

4. **Skin Irritation**

   DMSO can cause skin irritation or burning sensations at the site of application. To minimize this risk, it is important to properly clean and dry the area before applying DMSO. In case of severe skin irritation, discontinue usage and seek medical advice.

DMSO has been used as a therapeutic agent for various medical conditions, and its potential benefits are still being researched. It is important to follow proper precautions and inform your healthcare provider before using DMSO to ensure safe and effective usage. Always consult with your doctor if you experience any adverse effects while using this medication.

Common Mistakes to Avoid

While DMSO can provide potential benefits, there are some common mistakes that should be avoided to ensure safe and effective usage:

1. ***Overuse***: Excessive use of DMSO can lead to severe side effects, including skin irritation and systemic toxicity.
2. ***Ignoring Patch Tests***: Skipping patch tests can result in unexpected allergic reactions or skin damage.
3. ***Using High Concentrations***: Applying undiluted DMSO directly to the skin can cause burns and irritation.
4. ***Unsanitary Conditions***: Applying DMSO without proper hygiene can introduce contaminants into the body due to its transdermal properties.
5. ***Inconsistent Usage***: Inconsistent or improper use can diminish the benefits of DMSO and potentially worsen the condition being treated.

By following these tips and practices, you can safely and effectively utilize DMSO while minimizing risks.

Things to Do and to Avoid When Using Dimethyl Sulfoxide (DMSO)

Dimethyl sulfoxide (DMSO) is a versatile solvent with various applications, including pharmaceuticals, cryopreservation, and as a topical medication. However, it's essential to handle DMSO carefully due to its potent properties. Here are some things to do and not to do when using DMSO:

Things to Do

The following are some best practices to follow when using DMSO:

1. *Use Gloves*: Always wear gloves when handling DMSO to prevent it from penetrating the skin and carrying harmful substances into your body.
2. *Work in a Well-Ventilated Area*: Ensure that your workspace is well-ventilated to avoid inhaling fumes, which can cause respiratory irritation.
3. *Store Properly*: Keep DMSO in a cool, dry place, away from direct sunlight and heat sources. Make sure the container is tightly sealed.
4. *Label Clearly*: Clearly label any container holding DMSO to prevent accidental misuse or confusion with other substances.

5. ***Use Appropriate Containers***: Store DMSO in containers made from compatible materials (like glass or certain plastics) to avoid container degradation.
6. ***Wash Skin Immediately***: If DMSO comes into contact with your skin, wash the area thoroughly with soap and water to minimize absorption.
7. ***Use Dilutions Carefully***: When diluting DMSO, add it to the solvent slowly to minimize exothermic reactions that can cause heat and potential burns.

By following these best practices, you can safely and effectively use DMSO in various applications.

Things to Avoid

When working with DMSO, there are also some things you should avoid to prevent potential risks and hazards:

1. ***Avoid Contact with Contaminants***: Do not allow DMSO to contact other chemicals or contaminants, as it can carry these substances through the skin barrier.
2. ***Do Not Use on Broken Skin***: Avoid applying DMSO to broken or irritated skin to prevent rapid absorption and potential systemic effects.
3. ***Avoid Heat Sources***: Do not heat DMSO as it can become volatile and release harmful fumes.
4. ***Do Not Ingest***: Never ingest DMSO; it is intended for external use only and can be harmful if swallowed.

5. ***Avoid Using Metal Equipment***: DMSO can react with metals, so avoid using metal containers or tools when working with them.
6. ***Do Not Mix with Strong Oxidizers***: Avoid mixing DMSO with strong oxidizing agents, as this can lead to dangerous reactions.

By following these guidelines, you can safely handle DMSO and take advantage of its beneficial properties while minimizing risks.

Conclusion

Thank you for taking the time to read through this beginner's guide on DMSO. Your commitment to understanding DMSO demonstrates a proactive approach to gathering knowledge and making informed decisions. By now, you should have a comprehensive understanding of what DMSO is, its history, its various applications, and the necessary precautions one should take when handling it.

As you reflect on the information presented, it's essential to remember that DMSO, like many substances, requires careful consideration and a thoughtful approach. Understanding its properties and effects is crucial for anyone exploring its potential uses. Your interest in learning about DMSO is the first step toward making educated choices about whether or how to incorporate it into your practices.

One significant insight from this guide is the importance of personal experimentation under safe and controlled conditions. Individual responses to DMSO can vary significantly. Starting with small doses and observing your body's reactions allows you to gauge its effects accurately.

This personalized approach ensures that any use of DMSO aligns well with your unique needs and circumstances.

Staying informed about ongoing research and developments in the field of DMSO is equally important. Science and medical research are continually evolving, and new findings about DMSO's applications and effects are regularly published. Engaging with reputable sources of information and staying updated on current studies will further enhance your understanding and ability to make informed decisions.

It's also beneficial to consider the broader context of your health and wellness when exploring DMSO. Integrating it with other established health practices, such as maintaining a balanced diet, exercising regularly, and consulting healthcare professionals, can contribute positively to your overall well-being. While DMSO has a wide range of potential applications, it is not a standalone solution. A holistic approach to health, considering all aspects of your lifestyle, will provide the best foundation for any new practice you might consider.

The variety of applications for DMSO, from pain relief to its use as a solvent, highlights its versatility. However, this broad range of uses also underscores the necessity for correct application and adherence to safety guidelines. Misapplication or overuse can lead to adverse effects, so it is critical to follow recommended practices and seek expert advice when needed.

Your dedication to understanding DMSO reflects a commendable pursuit of knowledge. This proactive stance is essential when dealing with any substance that interacts closely with biological systems. By educating yourself, seeking credible information, and consulting with professionals, you empower yourself to make choices that best suit your personal needs and circumstances.

The journey you have started with DMSO is both exciting and responsible. The insights gained from this guide should serve as a foundation, helping you navigate future decisions with confidence and caution. Embrace the learning process, remain open to new information, and prioritize your health and safety at all times.

We appreciate your dedication to completing this guide and hope it serves as a valuable resource in your exploration of DMSO. Your commitment to understanding and applying these principles highlights a thoughtful and informed approach to health and wellness. Should you have further questions or wish to share your experiences, consider engaging with the larger community interested in DMSO. Your insights and discoveries could contribute to the collective understanding and promote safe practices.

FAQs

What is DMSO?

DMSO, short for Dimethyl Sulfoxide, is an organic sulfur compound that is used for its solvent properties and potential therapeutic benefits. It's known for its ability to penetrate the skin and other biological membranes.

What are the primary uses of DMSO?

DMSO is commonly used in medicine for reducing pain and inflammation, improving circulation, and promoting the healing of wounds and burns. It also finds use in veterinary medicine and as a solvent in various chemical reactions.

Is DMSO safe to use?

DMSO is generally considered safe when used properly, but it can cause side effects such as skin irritation, garlic-like breath, and allergic reactions. It's essential to use it under the guidance of a healthcare professional, especially for medical purposes.

How do I apply DMSO topically?

To apply DMSO topically, ensure the skin is clean and free from oils or lotions. Use a clean applicator such as a cotton ball or pad to apply a small amount of DMSO to the affected area. Allow it to dry completely. Always follow the dosage and application instructions provided by your healthcare provider or the product label.

Can DMSO be taken internally?

While some people use DMSO internally, it is generally not recommended without medical supervision due to potential risks and side effects. The FDA approves DMSO only for certain medical conditions and typically recommends external use.

What should I avoid when using DMSO?

Avoid using DMSO on broken or infected skin, combining it with other topical medications without professional advice, or exposing the treated area to direct sunlight. Always wash hands thoroughly after applying DMSO to prevent accidental contact with eyes or mucous membranes.

Where can I purchase DMSO?

DMSO can be purchased at health stores, online retailers, and pharmacies. When buying, ensure you select a high-quality, pharmaceutical-grade product to avoid contaminants and impurities.

References and Helpful Links

DiGiacinto, J. (2023b, May 16). What is DMSO? Healthline. https://www.healthline.com/health/what-is-dmso#:~:text=Dimethyl%20sulfoxide%20(DMSO)%20is%20a,reducing%20leakage%20during%20chemotherapy%20treatment.

Dimethyl sulfoxide | Fisher Scientific. (n.d.). https://www.fishersci.com/us/en/browse/80013630/dimethyl-sulfoxide?page=1

Akers, A. S. (2023, September 24). Can DMSO reduce arthritis symptoms? https://www.medicalnewstoday.com/articles/dmso-for-arthritis

Dludla, P. V., Nkambule, B. B., Mazibuko-Mbeje, S. E., Nyambuya, T. M., Silvestri, S., Orlando, P., Mxinwa, V., Louw, J., & Tiano, L. (2021). The impact of dimethyl sulfoxide on oxidative stress and cytotoxicity in various experimental models. In Elsevier eBooks (pp. 243–261). https://doi.org/10.1016/b978-0-12-819092-0.00025-x

Matthew. (2024, February 21). The Ultimate Guide to Dimethyl Sulfoxide (DMSO) [New - 2023]. Detox & Cure - Sea Moss | Shilajit | DMSO | Iron Fluorine. https://www.detoxandcure.com/the-ultimate-guide-to-dimethyl-sulfoxide-dmso/

Dimethyl sulfoxide - American Chemical Society. (n.d.). American Chemical Society. https://www.acs.org/molecule-of-the-week/archive/d/dimethyl-sulfoxide.html#:~:text=DMSO%20is%20a%20laboratory%20and,used%20solvent%20for%20chemical%20reactions.

Madsen, B. K., Hilscher, M., Zetner, D., & Rosenberg, J. (2019). Adverse reactions of dimethyl sulfoxide in humans: a systematic review. F1000Research, 7, 1746. https://doi.org/10.12688/f1000research.16642.2

www.ingramcontent.com/pod-product-compliance
Lightning Source LLC
LaVergne TN
LVHW012033060526
838201LV00061B/4591